Parenting Your Unborn Child

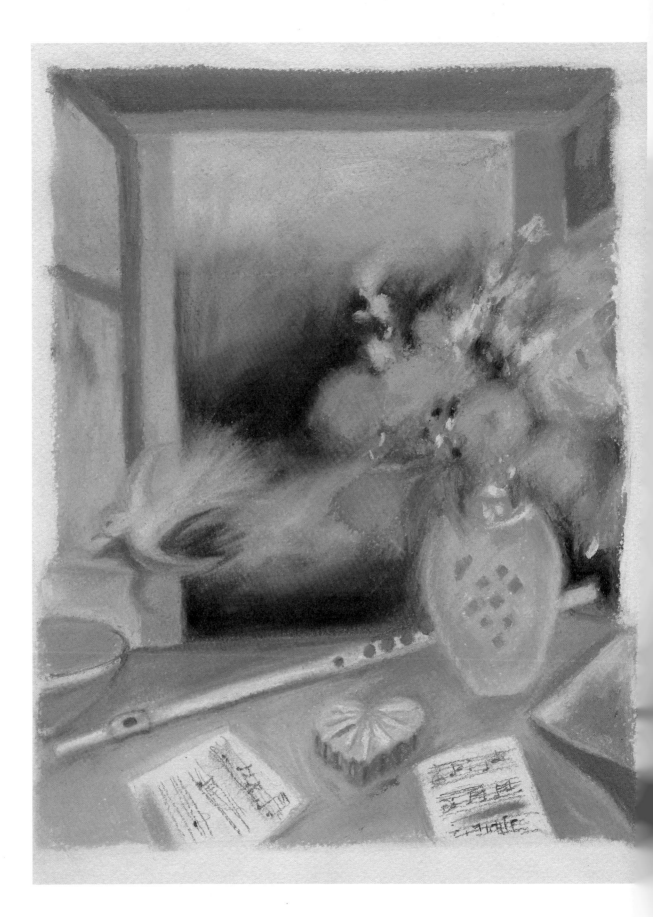

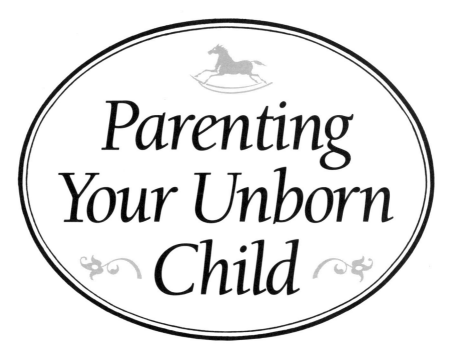

Parenting Your Unborn Child

A Practical Guide and Permanent Keepsake

Thomas R. Verny, M. D.

Doubleday Canada Limited, Toronto, Ontario

Design by The Dragon's Eye Press
Illustrations by Linda Montgomery
Editor: Colleen Darragh
Typesetting by Canadian Composition Inc.
Printed and bound in Canada by Friesen Printers

Canadian Cataloguing in Publication Data
Verny, Thomas
Parenting your unborn child

ISBN 0-385-25117-3

1. Baby books. 2. Fetus. 3. Childbirth.
4. Infants. I. Title.

HQ779.V47 1988 649'.1 C87-094097-X

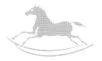

Contents

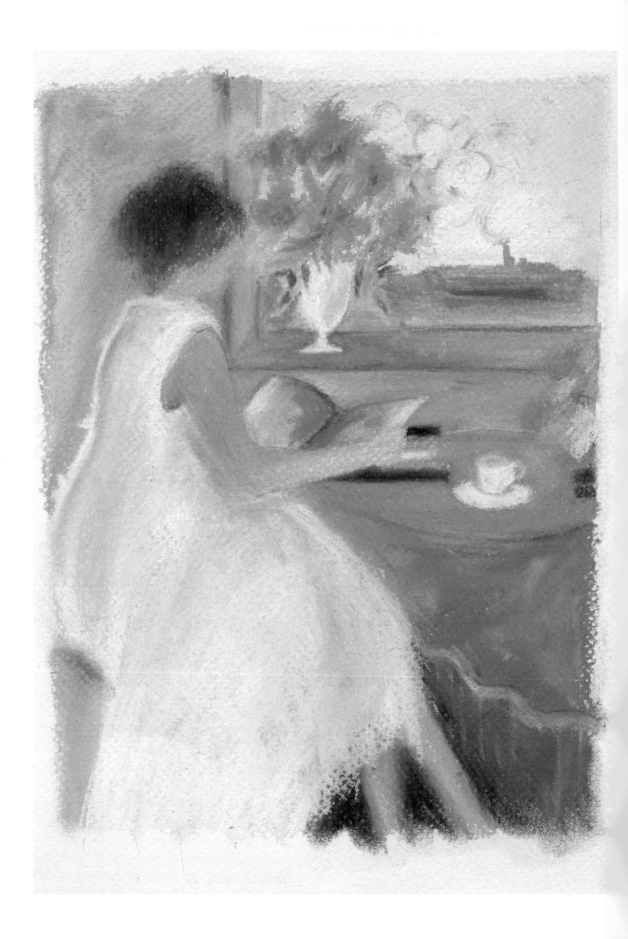

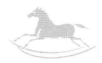

Introduction

MANY PEOPLE think of birth as marking the beginning of a person's life. To them, taking that first breath and uttering that first cry is like turning the light switch on in a darkened room. A flick of the wrist and there is light.

If you stop to think about it you quickly realize how false this popular notion really is.

We need to understand that one hour or one day or several weeks prior to birth, a child is not significantly different mentally from what she* is at birth. Very few babies are born exactly forty weeks after conception. Most are born days, weeks, sometimes even months prior to their "due date." Yet as long as they are not significantly premature they have no trouble adjusting to the outside world.

The mental apparatus of a baby is not suddenly thrown into gear with birth. All the complex tasks associated with living outside of the womb—like breathing, sucking, swallowing, touching, smelling, looking and listening—are the end result of mental work that started long before birth.

During the last two decades, due in large measure to the discoveries of scientists in the new field of pre- and peri-natal psychology, we have learned that the unborn child is a far more advanced being, both mentally and emotionally, than she was thought to be.

Through the use of advanced medical technology, it has become possible to study the unborn child undisturbed in her natural environment. Electrodes fastened to the scalp of the unborn baby allow one to obtain tracings of her brain waves. When soft optic fibers are inserted into the womb, one can observe the baby's movements and reactions to external stimuli. Ultrasound, fetal heart monitors and amniocentesis all contribute to a steady flow of information about the state of the unborn child.

*Throughout this book, "he" and "she" are used alternately when referring to the unborn or newborn child.

Some of the findings

By the fourth month after conception, the fetus will suck if his lips are stroked. If a bitter substance like iodine is introduced into the amniotic fluid, he will grimace and stop swallowing liquid.

At the same age, if a bright light is shone on the mother's abdomen the baby will gradually move his tiny hands up towards his eyes, shielding them. At five months, if a loud sound is made next to the mother the unborn child will raise his hands and cover his ears.

By the sixth month, the hearing system of the baby is perfectly developed. Because water is a better conductor of sound than air, the baby in the womb can hear very well, although with distortions.

Recording of the baby's brain waves at the beginning of the last trimester demonstrate that during sleep, the baby exhibits REM (Rapid Eye Movement) motions. In adults, REM sleep is almost always associated with dreaming. It follows, therefore that babies must be dreaming by the seventh month.

Studies of pregnant mothers show a correlation between their feelings about their pregnancies and the ease of their labors and deliveries. The health of their newborn infants is also connected to their attitudes towards pregnancy.

Milestones of fetal growth

Let me briefly review for you some of the major stages in development that lead from conception to birth. The mouth first opens on the 28th day (all times given here are post-conception). Stimulation of the baby's skin provokes slow, generalized movements of the head, trunk and extremities. At six weeks the earliest reflexes begin, which consist of sucking and grasping. Though the heart is still forming, it is already pumping blood. An ECG (electrocardiagram) tracing of the fetal heart would be very much like that of an adult heart. At this time, the fetus can make strong and brisk spontaneous movements.

By eight weeks, light stroking of the upper lip or the nose will cause the unborn infant to bend her neck and trunk away from the source of stimulation. EEG (electroencephalogram) tracings show brain wave activity similar to that of adults.

Between the ninth and twelfth weeks, babies are able to kick, turn their feet and curl their toes. They frown, purse their lips and open their mouths. Their primitive, empty lungs begin to expand and contract as though rehearsing for the day of birth. By the end of the third month, the baby measures approximately 3 inches (7.5 cm) and weighs about ½ an ounce (14 grams). Babies of the same age begin to show individual variations, particularly evident in their facial expressions.[1] When her eyelids are stroked now, the baby will squint instead of jerking her entire body back, as she did earlier. Stroking her lips will cause the fetus to respond by sucking.

At the end of the first trimester, the baby has developed all of her major systems and is virtually a functioning human being. However, she is still unable to survive independently.

The baby begins to suck her thumb and play with her umbilical cord in the fourth month. At this point in her development she is ready for conditional learning and, therefore, has a basic memory.

In the fifth month the baby will kick and turn, to the delight of her mother.

Periods of drowsiness and sleep alternate with periods of activity. Sleeping habits begin to appear.

By the sixth month, EEGs can differentiate not only between sleep and wakefulness, but also between REM sleep and non-REM sleep.

Dr. E. Wedenberg,[2] of the Karolinska Institute in Sweden, has researched pre-natal audiology. He notes that "after the 24th week it (the fetus) hears the mother's heart and intestinal sounds very intensely—or it should, for normal development."

The late Albert Liley,[3] research professor in prenatal physiology at Auckland University in New Zealand, similarly found that the mother's heartbeat and voice are audible to the fetus, and it is also likely that some light reaches the unborn child.

Hydrophones placed in the amniotic sac reveal that even ordinary conversation is clearly audible to the baby[4] against a background of sounds produced by the umbilical circulation, the steady thumping of the maternal heart and the rumblings of the maternal intestines.

Dr. Michele Clements,[5] a researcher in audiological medicine at the City of London Maternity Hospital, is convinced that what the baby hears—in the womb and after birth—can have a distinct bearing on the course of her life. She has further found that most babies like melodious music by composers such as Mozart or Vivaldi, but strongly reject the large orchestral pieces of Brahms and Beethoven. This theory can be easily tested by playing a certain musical selection close to the pregnant mother. If the mother feels her baby start to kick and to move about in a way that is unusual or painful, then this indicates her unborn child's discomfort. Rock music will produce this negative reaction, while musical selections that feature the flute, the violin or the harpsichord will have a calming effect.

Extensive studies leave no doubt that interaction between mother, father and the unborn—with all the consequences that it has for personality development—begins well before birth.

Because the unborn child from the sixth month after conception, if not before, is a feeling, sensing, aware and remembering being, and because of the intimate connection between her and her mother, everything that happens to the mother also in a sense happens to her baby. Everything that the mother eats, drinks and inhales is passed through her blood circulation into the body of her baby. That is why smoking, drinking alcohol or taking drugs should be avoided during pregnancy. What may be small amounts of these substances for the mother can be extremely harmful to the quickly growing baby, because of her size and general vulnerability.

Research during the past two decades has further demonstrated that maternal emotions are also transmitted to the unborn child.[6] The mother communicates with her child through three distinct channels. These usually work in concert, though sometimes one or the other is the dominant mode of communication.

If a pregnant mother experiences acute or chronic stress, her body manufactures stress hormones that reproduce in her baby the mother's own physiological and emotional state. We refer to this type of mother-child communication as physiological communication. Babies of mothers under stress are often premature, lower than average weight, hyperactive, irritable and colicky. On occasion some of these babies are born with thumbs sucked raw, while others a few days after birth are diagnosed as suffering from duodenal ulcers.

A second level of communication between the pregnant mother and her unborn child has been termed behavioral communication. This refers to the mother's activities with her baby such as patting her stomach, talking, singing, dancing and playing with her unborn infant. Of course, the father and other members of the family can all join in. The baby can respond by kicking and moving about. Just as the mother of a newborn quickly learns to distinguish the baby's cry of "Good morning, feed me" from "Hey, get that pin out of my behind!", so the pregnant mother can learn to differentiate between happy or distressed kicking. The important task for the mother-to-be is to learn to tune in to her baby, who very much wants to make contact with her.

Usually, behavioral communication is accompanied by psychological communication. By this I mean the baby's ability to register and respond to her mother's thoughts, feelings and spoken words. Babies pick up on the emotional charge that all spoken language carries. So when a mother strokes her baby through her abdomen and says something like "How are you, how is my wonderful baby?", the baby senses that she is loved and that makes her feel good. Many studies have shown that babies can tell whether their parents love them, reject them or feel ambivalent about them. We as adults thrive on love, praise and respect. Babies and children do, too.

So the more you can communicate with your unborn child and the calmer you are during your pregnancy, the more you will contribute to the healthy development of your baby.

This book is intended to help you develop your maternal and paternal instincts. By answering the questions raised here, you will become more aware of a variety of factors that may influence your baby's health and personality. You will learn to observe acutely and accurately the development of your unborn child which will enhance the enjoyment of your pregnancy. Most importantly, by learning to appreciate the sensitivity and sensibility of all babies, you will communicate with your own baby better than before, thus promoting the growth of a loving relationship between you and your unborn. This pre-natal "bonding" is the best foundation for your family's post-natal happiness.

As your child grows older, she will ask questions about her beginnings. This book will provide a complete record of her pre-natal life, birth and first twelve months. It will be an invaluable source of information for her. And should she, as an adult, wonder about some aspects of her personality, this book may help her to discover their origins. Some of her strengths, problems, talents, likes and dislikes may emerge in these pages.

In order to help you visualize your baby's growth, at the back of this book is a baby chart. By looking at this chart, you will know at a glance about what physical and mental progress your baby is making at any given point in your pregnancy.

One final piece of advice: Don't worry about being neat as you use this diary. You and your child will have more fun and reap more benefits from this book if you cram it full of photographs, newspaper clippings, lab reports, cards, telegrams and whatever else you find relevant. If the book starts bursting at the seams—just tie it up with ribbons and keep it in a safe place.

With best wishes for a happy pregnancy and a terrific baby,

Tom Verny, M.D.

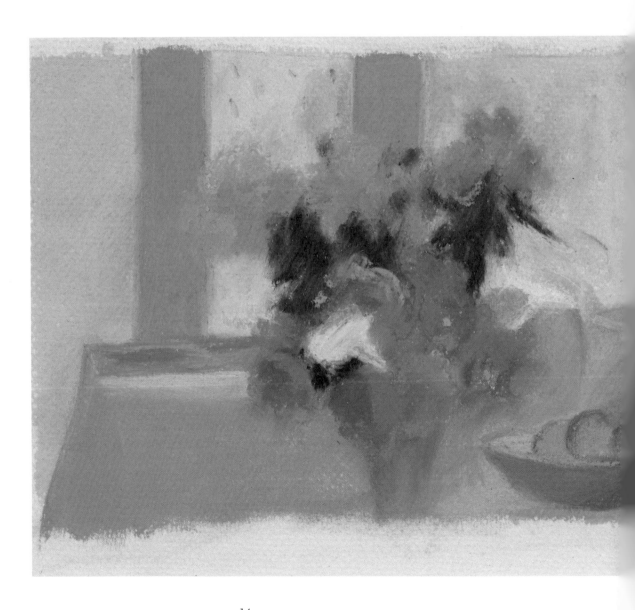

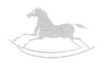

Preparing for Pregnancy

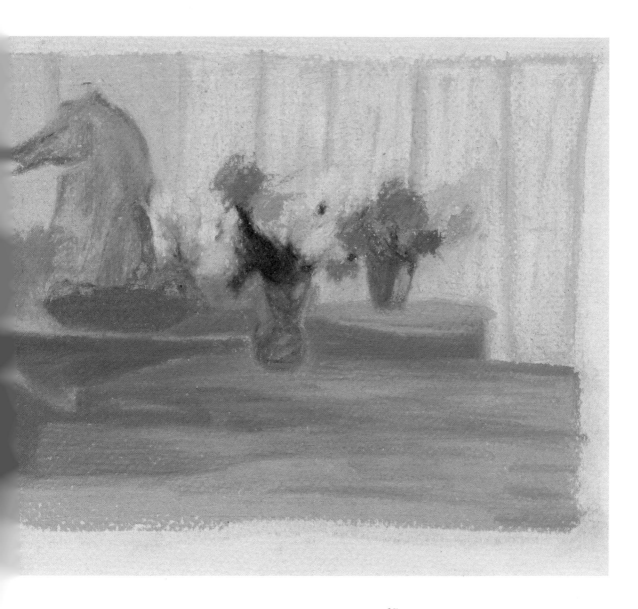

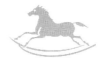

The Way You Were

Picture of mom before pregnancy

Picture of dad before pregnancy

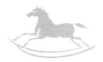

Making the Decision

Ideally how many children would you like to have?

_____

And your partner?

_____

Do you recall the first discussion you and your partner had about having children? Who said what?

_____
_____
_____
_____
_____
_____

Did you take any special measures to facilitate a healthy pregnancy? For example, did you stop smoking and drinking, change your diet, start a fitness program, etc.?

_____
_____
_____
_____
_____

Was there any particular person beside your partner whose advice you sought before you decided to start a family, such as a relative, friend, physician, counsellor or clergyman?

_____
_____

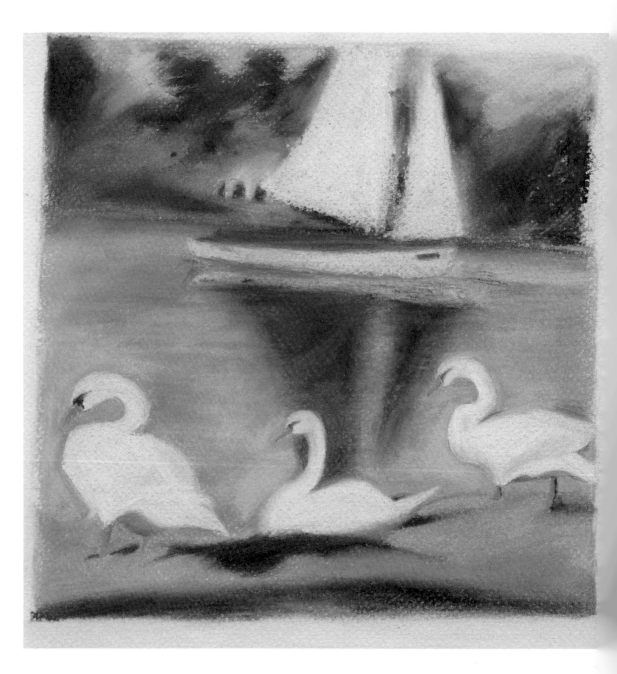

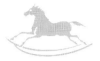

The First Days

When did you learn you were pregnant? How?

_____
_____
_____

Did you know deep down that you had conceived before the tests confirmed it?

_____
_____
_____

Did you have a dream or dreams that you interpreted as conception dreams or that in retrospect seem to relate to conception?

_____
_____
_____
_____
_____
_____
_____
_____

What was your initial reaction to finding out that you were pregnant?

_____
_____
_____
_____
_____
_____
_____

Your partner's reaction?

_____
_____
_____
_____
_____

For how long have you wanted this baby?

_____
_____
_____

Describe your moods in the days that followed your discovery of your pregnancy. What emotions did you feel? What were your dreams about?

_____
_____
_____
_____
_____
_____
_____
_____
_____
_____
_____
_____
_____
_____
_____

If this is not your first child, how do you think this pregnancy will differ from your previous one(s)?

_____
_____
_____
_____
_____
_____
_____
_____
_____
_____

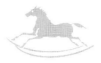

Pregnancy Milestones

You first visited the doctor on

_____

_____

His/her name was

_____

You were accompanied by

_____

_____

When did you first hear the baby's heartbeat by stethoscope?

_____

_____

Was your partner present?

_____

_____

How did you react when you heard the heartbeat?

_____

_____

_____

_____

_____

Did you have an ultrasound scan? If so, when?

_____

_____

Place a picture of your ultrasound scan here. (You can request a copy from your doctor.)

How did you feel when you saw your baby on the screen during the ultrasound scan? Was your partner with you?

_____
_____
_____
_____
_____
_____
_____
_____

Does anything about the baby's position or features provide clues to your child's personality or appearance?

_____
_____
_____
_____
_____
_____
_____
_____

Are you scheduled for other tests, e.g., amniocentesis, chorionic villi sampling (cvs), additional ultrasonography?

_____
_____
_____
_____
_____
_____
_____

Did your baby's movements change at all while the testing was performed?

_____
_____
_____
_____
_____
_____
_____

When did you first feel truly pregnant—convinced that you were carrying a child?

_____
_____
_____
_____
_____
_____
_____

When did you first feel the baby move? Where were you? Was the activity vigorous, gentle, momentary, lengthy?

_____
_____
_____
_____
_____
_____
_____
_____
_____
_____

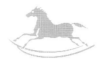

Baby's Habits

When was the first time you felt the baby kicking?

_____

Does your baby ever get hiccups?

_____

Baby's favorite position

_____
_____
_____

Baby's favorite activity

_____
_____
_____

When is your baby most active?

_____

Least active?

_____

Has the baby awakened you in the night because of strong kicks or other behavior?

_____
_____

Does your baby sleep at the same time as you do?

_____
_____

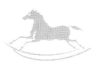

Parents' Health and Habits

Your health during your pregnancy

_____
_____
_____
_____

Your partner's health during your pregnancy

_____
_____
_____
_____

Favorite activities during your pregnancy

_____
_____
_____
_____
_____
_____
_____
_____

Favorite foods during your pregnancy

_____
_____
_____
_____
_____
_____
_____
_____

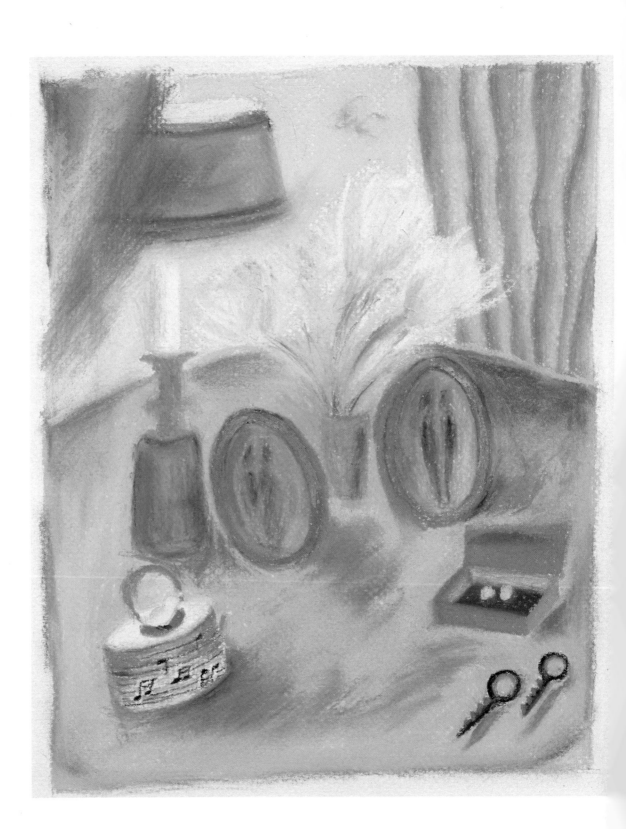

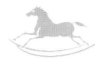

Parents' Feelings and Relationship

*T*HIS SECTION focuses on the mental and emotional state of the mother and father during pregnancy. As you read on, keep in mind that fleeting worries or anxieties are a normal part of pregnancy. They have no adverse effect on the baby. In fact, a certain amount of anxiety stimulates the mental faculties of the baby. On the other hand, deep, persistent negative feelings, prolonged depression or chronic stress may be harmful to him.

It's very important for babies to feel wanted. If this pregnancy came as a total surprise to you and you feel ambivalent about having a baby, the important thing is to talk about your feelings with someone you trust. You can do so with the father of the child, a friend or a mental health professional. What matters is that you don't pretend to yourself that you feel fine when in reality you are quite upset.

Your relationship with your mate will make a difference to your baby. Every study done on this subject shows that a good relationship positively correlates with an easy pregnancy and the birth of a healthy child. Similarly, the pregnant mother's relationship with her own parents—particularly her mother— seems to be an important factor in the pregnancy equation. If your parents chronically criticized you and if you have a poor rapport with them now, then this may unconsciously cause you undue strain during your pregnancy. So ask yourself: how did my parents make me feel about me, about my body, about having and raising children? Share your thoughts and feelings with your partner and you will see how many helpful insights such conversations can yield.

A word about stress. Remember that stress is a very subjective phenomenon. What may be perceived as stressful to one person will not necessarily affect another individual in that way. Too often doctors, well-meaning relatives or friends make global pronouncements that produce more harm than good. For example, everybody (myself included) will advise pregnant mothers against smoking. But, if quitting smoking turns you into a nervous wreck, makes you unbearably irritable and means that you gain ten pounds in a week, you may be better off to cut down on your habit, rather than stopping altogether.

Similarly, the question about working and pregnancy often arises. How long into the pregnancy should a woman work? My answer is that she ought not to work during the last two months. However, there are many women who genuinely enjoy their jobs and staying at home with nothing to do would drive these mothers-to-be up the wall. Obviously, working for as long as they feel like it will be beneficial for such women.

What is happening around you during your pregnancy? Have there been notable family events, career changes, moves, travel?

_____
_____
_____
_____
_____
_____
_____
_____
_____
_____
_____
_____
_____
_____
_____
_____
_____
_____
_____
_____
_____

Is your pregnancy a relaxed period in your life or is it causing you some stress? Do you notice changes in your personality right now?

_____
_____
_____
_____
_____
_____
_____
_____
_____
_____

Is your relationship with your mate undergoing any changes?

_____

_____

_____

_____

_____

_____

_____

_____

_____

_____

_____

_____

_____

_____

_____

_____

_____

_____

_____

_____

_____

_____

_____

_____

_____

_____

_____

_____

_____

_____

_____

_____

_____

_____

_____

_____

_____

_____

_____

_____

_____

_____

_____

Place a few pictures here of yourself at different stages of your pregnancy.

Picture of family during pregnancy—mom, dad, brothers, sisters, grandparents

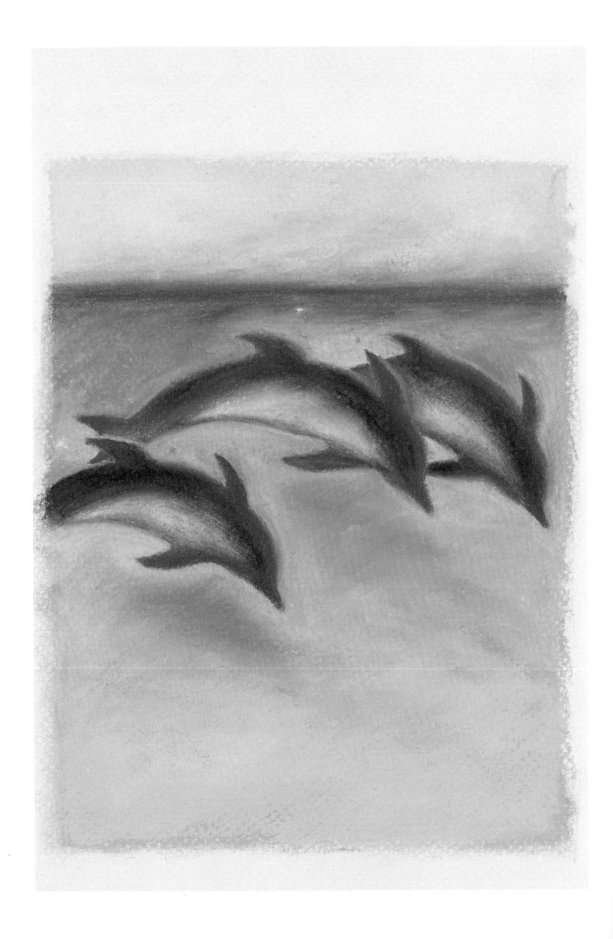

Communicating
with Your Baby

ANTHONY DeCASPER, professor of psychology at the University of North Carolina, has been researching fetal perception and memory for the past ten years. He has conducted a remarkable series of experiments. First, he demonstrated that newborns can pick out their mothers' voices from among other female voices.[7] DeCasper wondered, however, if babies might not just prefer a familiar voice to an unfamiliar one heard after birth. These infants were then tested with a non-nutritive nipple hooked up to a tape recorder to see if they preferred their fathers' voices to that of other men's. (By changing the rhythm of their sucking, the babies could switch the taped voices.) They did not. However, after a few weeks they were retested and they did opt for their fathers' voices.

Next, DeCasper rigged up his "suck-o-meter" in such a way that infants could choose between listening to a taped maternal heartbeat and a taped male voice. The majority of babies favored a tape recording of the heartbeat.[8]

Finally, a group of pregnant mothers was asked to tape record their reading of two different children's stories: "The Cat in the Hat" and "The King, the Mice and the Cheese." During the last six and a half weeks of their pregnancy, half the group was asked to read story A twice a day and the other half read story B. When the babies were born, the researchers offered them a choice between the two stories. Within a few hours after birth, eleven of the twelve newborns adjusted their sucking rhythm to hear the familiar story as opposed to the new story.[9]

These data provide the first direct evidence that not only does the unborn hear and recognize his mother's voice, but also—and this is the real shock—he remembers the words!

Rene Van de Carr is an obstetrician in Hayward, California, who has applied the new knowledge about the incredible mind power of babies to a program of pre-natal stimulation which he calls, tongue-in-cheek, the Pre-natal University. Here he encourages pregnant mothers not only to talk, play music and read stories to their unborn children, but also to associate words with actions. For example, he advises a mother to say "pat, pat, pat" while patting the baby's back or "rub, rub, rub" while rubbing her abdomen. The pre-natally stimulated babies are generally described as quick, very adaptive and socially aware.

What does this new research mean for you, as expectant parents? Simply this: talk to your unborn baby as much as possible, whenever you feel like it. Speak in a soft voice. Your partner and any other members of the family can join in. Don't be shy or self-conscious. What you say is not as important as how you say it. "It's raining today and I'm thinking of you," will earn you the Pulitzer Prize from your baby. Feel free to read children's stories, nursery rhymes or poems. Avoid violent subjects and overly dramatic readings. Remember that children like repetition, so one or two stories a few times a day will be sufficient.

After the birth of your child, try your own experiment. Does your newborn, like the infants in Dr. DeCasper's study, prefer the familiar tale to a story that he has never heard?

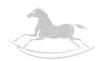

Talking to the Baby

When did you start to talk to your unborn baby?

_____

When did your partner start?

_____

What do you say?

_____
_____
_____

Do you read to the baby? If so, what?

_____
_____
_____

Does anyone else talk to the baby (e.g., another child)?

_____
_____
_____

Do any words or phrases produce a predictable response?

_____
_____
_____

Is there a difference in how the baby reacts to your voice or your partner's?

_____
_____
_____

Touching the Baby

We know that by the seventh week after conception, the baby responds to tactile stimulation. At twelve weeks she can kick, turn her feet and curl her toes. At sixteen weeks she begins to suck her thumb. So, the sense of touch is obviously developed very early, and is necessary to the well-being of the baby. She uses it to explore her aquatic universe as well as to comfort herself. Thus thumb-sucking not only calms the baby but also helps her to develop her coordination and to strengthen her jaw and cheek muscles.

Like all living beings, babies like to be touched. You can discover this for yourself after the baby grows big enough for you to feel her kicks. At this point, just start stroking your abdomen gently from below to your belly button. You will quickly observe that your baby will stop kicking and relax. By about the seventh month of pregnancy, you will know the positions of your baby's head and feet. Stroke firmly and repetitively from her head towards her toes. This is thought to accelerate the development of her peripheral nervous system.

More importantly, your massage helps you to make contact with your baby and, like talking and playing music, enhances the baby's feeling of being loved. This in turn contributes to the baby's development of a strong and healthy sense of self-esteem. It is important to realize that even our egos have their beginnings in the womb.

Towards the end of your pregnancy you can actually play with your unborn. Push one finger into one side of your abdomen and then push in on the other side. Repeat this routine a few times and you will be amazed to find that your baby will pick up your pattern and push against your hand. (Of course, she can only do so if her back is lined up against your back.) Many mothers have told me that touching their babies' hands through the abdominal wall was the most thrilling event of their pregnancies.

Dr. Susan Ludington-Hoe reports on a study of 120 babies who were given 100 minutes of extra skin-to-skin stroking over the first three days of life. These babies gained weight faster and performed motor movements earlier than a

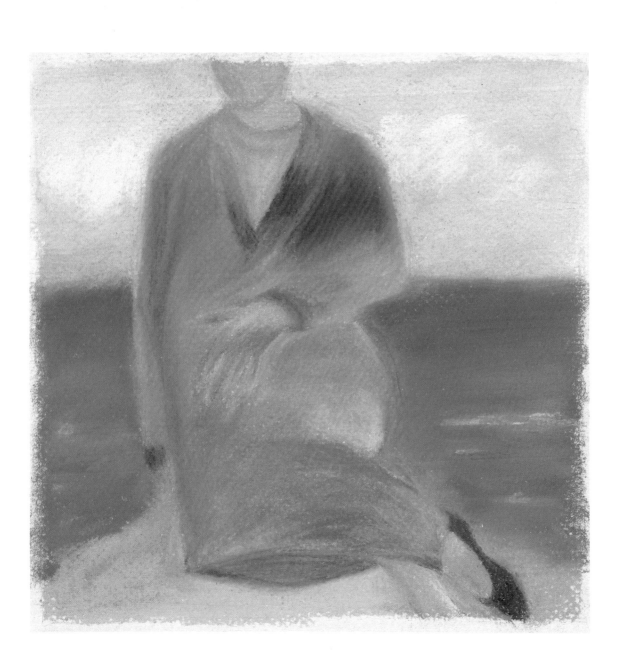

group of babies who did not receive the extra contact.[10] Consequently, it is important to continue to touch the baby, to stroke her and to massage her after the birth also. Do so from the head downwards and from the center of the body towards the toes and fingertips. Gently massaging the neck and shoulders and stroking the forehead is particularly soothing.

Fathers, for some reason, like to tickle their babies and to throw them up in the air or make motions as if they were going to do so. Please don't. Tickling annoys babies and sudden and violent changes to their positions frightens them at this early age. Furthermore, an abrupt jerking of the head may injure a baby's neck.

Do you prefer any particular time of day or night to touch the baby, rub your tummy or massage the baby?

_____
_____
_____

Does your partner?

_____
_____
_____

Does anyone else make physical contact with your baby?

_____
_____
_____

What games do you play with the baby?

_____
_____
_____
_____
_____

How does the baby respond?

_____
_____
_____
_____
_____

Music and the Baby

Mothers have known about the effect of music on unborn children for generations. Scientists, however, are just beginning to discover it. Experiments with animals[11] and human fetuses[12] have clearly shown that sound is transmitted through body walls and amniotic fluid with about a 30 decibel loss in intensity. Human infants respond to sound by six months after conception.[13]

How can we be sure of this? Well, it's really not very difficult. First, you observe the baby's movements through the abdomen and note his heart rate, (with a stethoscope) thus establishing a baseline of activity. Then you play music close to the mother. If the baby shifts his position and starts to move his hands and feet in rhythm to the music and his pulse quickens or, with particularly soothing music, he slows down or stops moving entirely and his pulse slackens—then you know he is listening and reacting to the music.

Hundreds of women have told me about their experiences with music during pregnancy. The one common denominator to all these accounts is that whatever pieces of music these mothers played and whatever songs they sang to their unborn children provoked a very positive reaction in their babies after birth. The familiar music seemed to capture the attention of their infants, as well as relax them.

Because of its calming effect on their children, mothers found this "pre-natal music" particularly helpful when their children were cranky, overtired or feverish.

Donald Shetler, a professor of music education at the University of Rochester, has been studying the effect of music during pregnancy on infant development. He has found that infants exposed to music while in the womb show a remarkable ability to imitate sound and respond to it after birth, in comparison to babies who have not had "pre-natal musical stimulation...."[14]

Professional musicians such as Yehudi Menuhin, Artur Rubinstein, Boris Brott and many others—as well as countless non-musicians—feel strongly that their musical abilities, talents or preferences started in the womb.

I personally recommend playing music during pregnancy. It should be music that the pregnant mother likes, and it should be calming rather than exciting. The only type of music that should definitely be avoided is hard rock (acid rock, heavy metal, etc.). Listen to the music with the best equipment possible, while doing nothing else. Listen to each piece closely, for ten minutes or so. Make sure that you are comfortably sitting or reclining in pleasant surroundings.

If you are like most expectant mothers I know, after reading the above you will resolve to follow my advice but there will always be other more pressing matters that will somehow prevent you from taking the time out for yourself. So I urge you to get into a daily routine as set and fixed as brushing your teeth. Choose two times during the day—for example, after lunch and before bedtime—that you can listen to your "pregnancy tape" undisturbed.

When you do, you will enjoy a number of benefits. First, by reserving two ten-minute periods for doing "nothing but listening to music" you will interrupt your busy schedule of activities and relax. You can also enhance the stress-relieving advantage of good music—I recommend the slow movements of baroque and classical composers like Vivaldi, Mozart, Haydn, etc.*—by breathing slowly and evenly and allowing the music to enter your body (without analyzing the music in your head). If you feel like it, tap your feet, sway or dance to the music. As you do that, you will find yourself relaxing and that's an excellent experience for you and your baby.

A second benefit of music is that it will stimulate your baby's mind. The brain is like a muscle, the more you use it the better it functions. You will recall the research described earlier that indicated the desirable effects of pre-natal stimulation. Though our aim should never be to produce little Mozarts or Einsteins, depriving our babies of the opportunity to exercise their brains seems like a terrible waste of their natural potential. So think of music as food for the intellectual development of your baby.

Lastly, and most importantly, the music serves as an emotional bridge between the mother and her unborn child. This occurs because while she listens to the music, the mother's mind will automatically shift to thoughts about her baby. The pregnant mother will try to "see" the baby and will accompany this picture with thoughts or spoken wishes for the health and well-being of the unborn child. With each day she will grow closer to her baby and get to know him better. In this way the mother learns to love her infant and the child feels this love long before birth.

I also recommend that you play your pregnancy tape during your labor, to help you, your baby and your birth attendants to relax. After the baby is born, continue to play the music to him when you want to calm him, for example, at bedtime.

*A recent recording of classical music designed for the pregnant mother specifically is *Love Chords*, available from A & M Records of Canada and from Nate Systems, Salt Lake City, Utah.

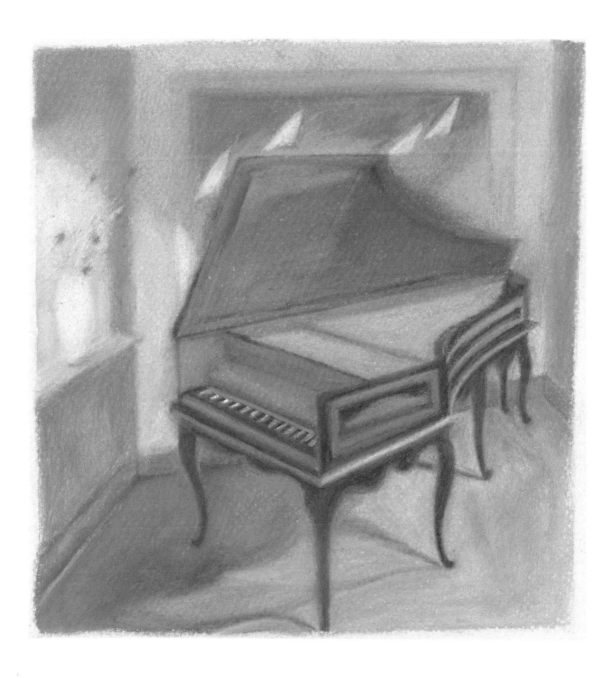

Describe the type of music you play during your pregnancy.

_____
_____
_____
_____
_____
_____
_____
_____
_____

Songs you and your partner sing

_____
_____
_____
_____
_____
_____
_____
_____
_____

What time of day do you hold your music sessions? Where do you listen?

_____
_____
_____
_____
_____

Baby's reactions to music

_____
_____
_____
_____
_____

Baby's favorite music

_____
_____
_____
_____
_____

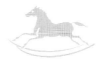

Getting to Know Your Unborn Baby

Record your first impressions about your unborn baby's personality, appearance, sex.

_____
_____
_____
_____
_____
_____
_____
_____
_____
_____
_____
_____
_____

Have you visualized your baby?

_____
_____
_____
_____
_____
_____

Have you meditated about the baby?

_____
_____
_____
_____
_____
_____

Do you feel that your baby has tried to communicate with you? How?

_____

_____

_____ _____

_____

_____

_____

_____

_____

What kind of connection do you feel between you and your unborn baby?

_____

_____

_____

_____

_____

_____

_____

_____

_____

_____

_____

_____

_____

_____

_____

_____

_____

_____

_____

_____

_____

_____

_____

_____

_____

_____

_____

_____

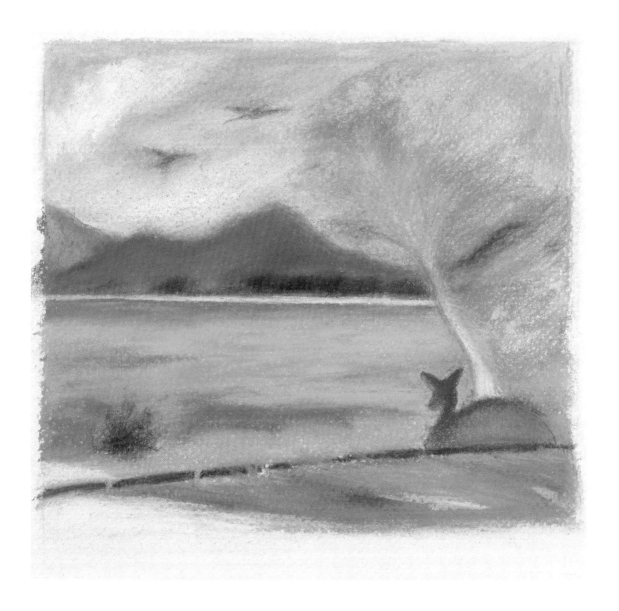

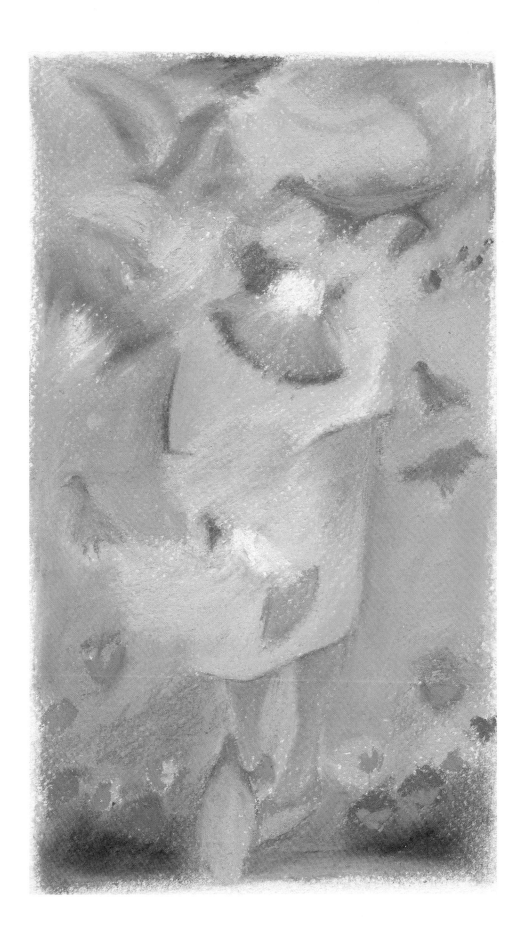

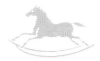

Dreaming during Pregnancy

*T*HOUGH MANY PEOPLE do not remember their dreams, everyone has them—four or five a night, one about every ninety minutes. Freud called dreams "the royal road to the unconscious" and that assessment is as true today as it was in his day. Dream images reveal how the unconscious views what is going on in our waking lives and in our bodies. While Freud thought of dreams as largely an outlet for repressed sexual and aggressive drives, most clinicians today (while not denying the validity of his view) consider dreams as serving a positive and healing function as well. In other words, while the dream may express certain hidden conflicts, it may also call the dreamer's attention to unrecognized talents or neglected aspects of personality that require attention if the individual is to continue to grow and mature.

In a study that investigated the relationship of dreams to childbirth, researchers[15] found that women who experienced anxiety in more than 80 percent of their dreams delivered their babies in less than average time. Women who had anxiety in only 25 percent of their dreams took the longest time to deliver, while women who fell into the middle range in their reports of anxiety in dreams were also intermediate in the length of their labors. The researchers concluded that the pregnant women who reported long dreams with anxious themes of childbirth were "psychologically immunizing" themselves in their dreams.

Because dreams can be an important learning experience, we should pay close attention to them—particularly during pregnancy. You can improve your ability to recall dreams by reminding yourself every night, before drifting off to sleep, to have a dream.

Keep this book next to your bed and as soon as you wake up, jot down your dream on the following pages with as much detail as possible. Then during the day, try to find some time to reread your dream and to reflect on it. If any of your dreams concern you, discuss them with a psychotherapist who is knowledgeable about dreams. You may also wish to start a dream group for pregnant mothers where, through mutual sharing of your dream lives, much can be learned.

Add your personal reactions to the dreams, along with conversations you may have had about them. Note your partner's dreams about your unborn child too.

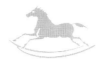

Dreams
During Pregnancy

For easy reference, try to date each dream and to give it a title (for example, "The Teddy Bear and the Whistle," January 15, 1988). If you run out of space, add more pages.

Title _____

Date _____

Dream _____

_____

_____

_____

_____

_____

_____

_____

_____

_____

_____

Title _The Easy Birth_

Date _Feb 11 /93_

Dream _I am pregnant and so is someone else (perhaps Elanor) We both get not as large as I am now. When the baby drops we get much smaller more comfy. The other person has her baby first. It is an easy birth and the baby is beautiful with an unearthly glow. It is a boy. I have an easy birth and it is a very beautiful girl with the same spiritual glow. The babys are at some point taken out of a paper bag which is when the glow is noticed. There is a nice design of vertical lines coming from the centre of the bag._

Title _____

Date _____

Dream _____

_____

_____

_____

_____

_____

_____

_____

_____

_____

_____

_____

Title _____

Date _____

Dream _____

_____

_____

_____

_____

_____

_____

_____

_____

_____

_____

_____

_____

_____

Title _____

Date _____

Dream _____

_____

_____

_____

_____

_____

_____

_____

_____

_____

_____

_____

Title _____

Date _____

Dream _____

_____

_____

_____

_____

_____

_____

_____

_____

_____

_____

_____

_____

Title _____

Date _____

Dream _____

_____

_____

_____

_____

_____

_____

_____

_____

_____

_____

_____

_____

_____

Title _____

Date _____

Dream _____

_____

_____

_____

_____

_____

_____

_____

_____

_____

_____

_____

Title _____

Date _____

Dream _____

_____

_____

_____

_____

_____

_____

_____

_____

_____

_____

_____

Title _____

Date _____

Dream _____

_____

_____

_____

_____

_____

_____

_____

_____

_____

_____

_____

_____

Title _____

Date _____

Dream _____

_____

_____

_____

_____

_____

_____

_____

_____

_____

_____

Title _____

Date _____

Dream _____

_____

_____

_____

_____

_____

_____

_____

_____

_____

_____

_____

Title _____

Date _____

Dream _____

_____

_____

_____

_____

_____

_____

_____

_____

_____

_____

_____

_____

_____

Title _____

Date _____

Dream _____

_____

_____

_____

_____

_____

_____

_____

_____

_____

_____

_____

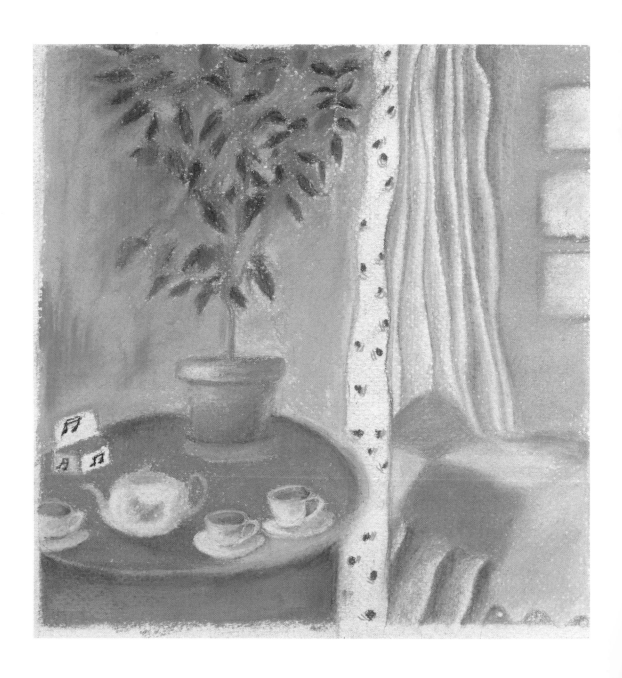

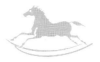

Preparation for Birth

*E*VERY LARGE URBAN CENTER now offers a great variety of childbirth preparation classes. Some of these are hospital-affiliated. Others are given by large organizations such as the Lamaze Association or the International Childbirth Education Association, while still others are run by individual midwives.

Investigate several before making your choice. Look for a course that covers more than just the nuts and bolts of pregnancy and delivery. One that deals with the emotional aspects of this period will be especially helpful. Ideally, share these classes with the father of your child. If he is not available and if he does not plan to be present at the birth, arrange to be accompanied at the classes by a close friend who can provide you with emotional support during your pregnancy and the baby's birth.

Choosing a doctor is of course crucial to a good birth experience. More and more obstetricians and family physicians who deliver babies are becoming aware, happily, of the importance of a non-medicated, non-interventionist birth for both mother and child. Do not hesitate to interview your doctor about his or her philosophy and delivery practice.

The model doctor will reassure you that he or she will be present at the birth (some doctors are on call only every third day, for example); that you will not be induced as a convenience; that you will not be given painkillers unnecessarily; that forceps will not be used unless absolutely mandatory; and that an episiotomy will not be performed routinely. Your partner and your birth attendant should be allowed to be present. Ask your doctor if you can use a cassette tape recorder with your prenatal music tape during labor and delivery. Be sure that the doctor will not cut the baby's cord prematurely. Will your doctor agree to let you hold the baby? Ask about the doctor's policy on silver nitrate for the newborn's eyes. These are only necessary if a mother has gonorrhea, yet they are given routinely in most hospitals. Is your doctor willing to skip them, so your baby can be spared discomfort? Silver nitrate also blurs the newborn's vision thus interfering with bonding.

In this space, record your choice of pre-natal classes—where they are held, your instructor's name and the dates that you attend.

_____
_____
_____
_____
_____
_____
_____
_____
_____
_____
_____
_____
_____
_____
_____
_____
_____
_____
_____
_____
_____
_____

Who accompanies you?

_____

Do you enjoy the classes?

_____
_____
_____
_____

If you had to summarize your feelings about your pregnancy right now in a word or two, what would you say?

_____
_____

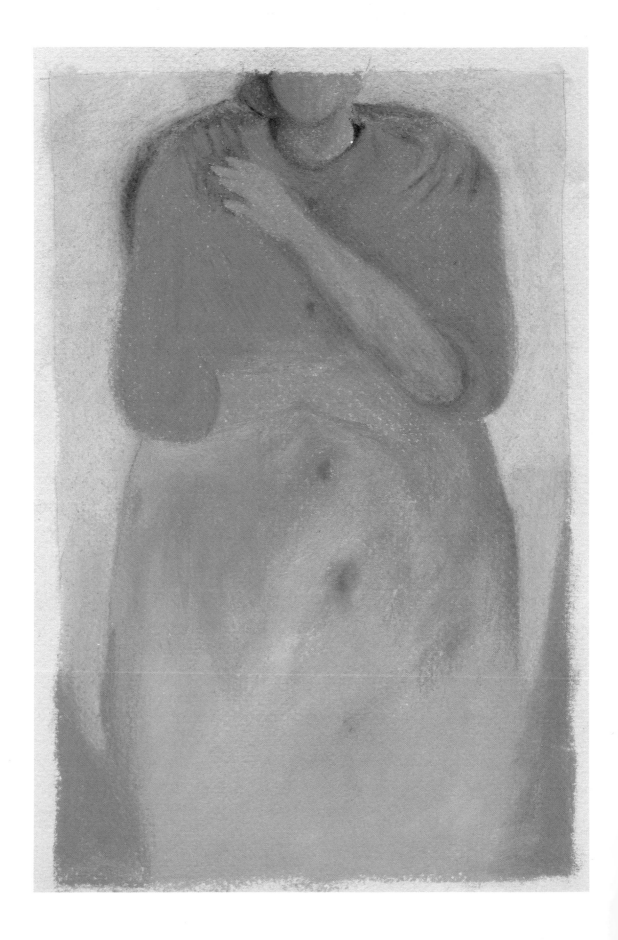

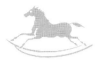

The Birth

DURING THE LAST CENTURY birthing has moved from the home into the hospital. The hospital is run by doctors and nurses who are trained to treat sick people. Consequently, a person who occupies a bed in the hospital is likely to be treated by the staff as an ill patient. In this simple way, without anyone giving it much thought and with the best of intentions by health professionals, the natural process of birth has over the years been transformed into a medical/surgical procedure.

What are the consequences of this "hospitalization" of birth for the pregnant woman? In the worst case the following things may happen.

On admission the pregnant woman receives a name tag with a number. Then she is asked to disrobe and change into a hospital gown which leaves her totally exposed from the back, increasing her feeling of vulnerability. She is immediately confined to her room and then has a variety of nurses, interns and residents examine her. Gradually, the pregnant woman's sense of individuality and her self-esteem are eroded.

The pregnant mother finds herself in an unfamiliar place where she has to obey peculiar rules enforced by strangers.

Because the staff are experts and the patient is not, the pregnant woman is made to feel as if others know more about her body than she does. Moreover, the staff behave as if her body had become theirs, to do with as they please.

As the pain and the anxiety mount, the staff, in their attempts to be helpful, offer her painkillers. These in turn will slow down contractions even more, until the doctors increasingly intervene and apply a variety of measures to speed delivery—from forceps and episiotomy to induction of labor with Pitocin to a caesarean section. Then the mother is encouraged to be grateful for the wonderful care she has received.

Today, hospitals, obstetricians, peri-natal nurses and other health professionals involved in birthing are changing all this. There is a genuine attempt being made to respect the emotional needs of the pregnant mother and her family. However, it is a fact of life that hospitals, like other large institutions,

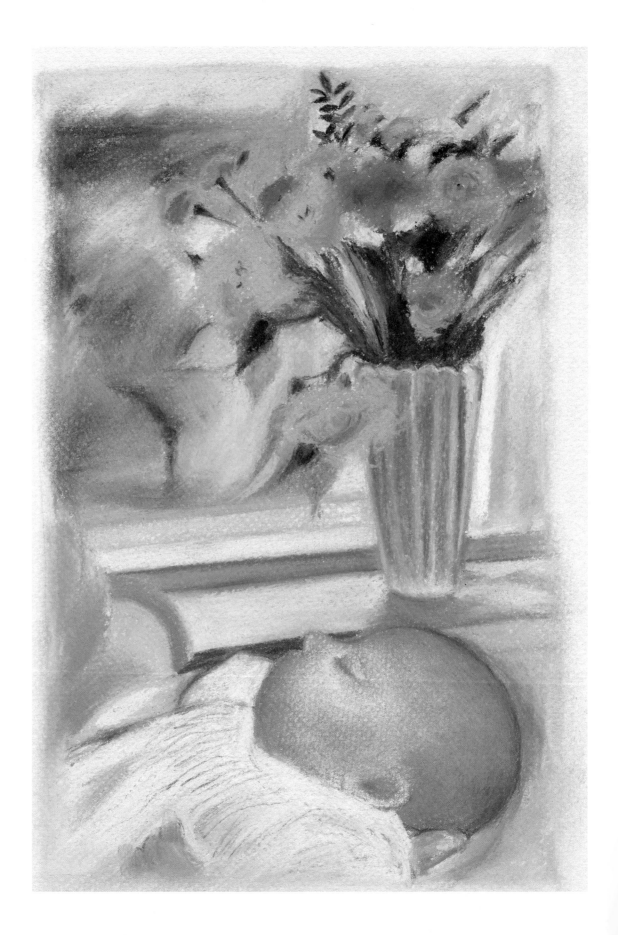

have their own agendas which may be different from those of the consumer. It is therefore important for you to be well informed, to know what kind of obstetrical care you want and then to insist on receiving it.

Though I believe that, from a psychological standpoint, the best place for a child to be born is at home, most studies seem to indicate that home births are not as safe as hospital births. A good compromise, then, is to give birth either in a birth center that is properly staffed and equipped for emergencies, or in a birthing room in a hospital. I would recommend that the woman in labor be accompanied by her spouse and a midwife or birth attendant. While a pregnant mother by herself does not stand a chance of prevailing against doctors or nurses who want to interfere with her labor, her wishes are far more likely to be respected if she is accompanied by one or two other people.

Taking into consideration the results of the latest research and of interviews with pregnant mothers, an ideal birth should provide as many of the following conditions as possible:

• supportive obstetrical staff with a "high-touch" instead of a "hi-tech" orientation

• a birthing room that is comfortable, home-like and quiet

• the freedom to walk around throughout your labor and to give birth in any position you prefer

• the presence of your spouse and birth attendant, as well as any friends or family you wish to include

• no fetal heart monitors, drugs, episiotomies or forceps unless they are necessary and you agree to their use

• access to your pre-natal music played during labor and delivery

• dim lights and an atmosphere of unhurried calm during the birth process

• placement of the baby on your chest right after birth

• immediate father/baby contact (the father can hold the newborn and give her a bath, if possible)

• no silver nitrate drops for baby's eyes

Following the birth, ask that the baby stay with you in your room if both of you are healthy. Then leave the hospital as soon as you can, go home and enjoy your baby.

Your Experience of the Birth Process

Length of labor
Water broke at 7:55am April 5 - born 3:25 am April 6   19

Place of birth: home, hospital, birthing room?
Birthing Room, Campbell River Hospital

Exact time of birth
3:25 AM April 6 1993

Birth attendants: midwife, doctors, nurses?
Alexander, Brenda Dempsey Kathie Landry
Wendy Walsh   Dr Steve Martin
Mary   Jane

Was your baby's father present?
Yes! Yes! Yes! Very Present (most of the time)

Was a fetal heart monitor used?
No

Were any painkillers, anesthetics or forceps used?
No

Did you have any surgery (caesarean, episiotomy)?
No

Did you play music? If so, what pieces?
Windham Hill
Annie Lennox

Did anyone film the birth or take photos?

Kathie Videod + took birth pictures
Wendy Videod while Kathie took pictures

Were you able to hold the baby immediately? How much time did you spend
with your baby after delivery?

Yes - Steve put Serena up on my belly
immediately after she was born. She was
purpulish + kind of flaccid-but very bright eyed

Was the father of help to you?

Alexander was a great emotional
support to me. He was very excited
and cried while Serena jumped out and when
he first held Serena.

Did the father cut the cord or give the baby a bath?

Alexander cut the cord while Serena was
on my chest

Describe the labor and birth. Be as specific as possible. Include a physical
description of the labor and birthing rooms and record any conversations you
can recall, particularly between you and your partner.

What was your reaction when you first saw your child?

_____

_____

_____

_____

_____

How did your newborn react at the moment of delivery, and in the minutes that followed?

_____

_____

_____

_____

_____

_____

_____

_____

_____

_____

How did you feel when you first held your baby?

_____

_____

_____

_____

_____

_____

_____

_____

_____

_____

What was the mood in the delivery room?

_____

_____

_____

_____

_____

How long did you stay in the hospital?

_____

_____

Were you pleased with your hospital care?

_____
_____
_____
_____
_____

Describe your baby's first few days (whether in the hospital or at home) and the experience of caring for the newborn.

_____
_____
_____
_____
_____
_____
_____
_____
_____
_____
_____

In the space below, place the first photo of your baby.

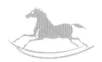

A Birth Record

Apgar score _____ Weight _____ Height _____

Complexion _____
_____

Color of hair _____
_____

Color of eyes and eyebrows _____
_____

Shape of head _____
_____

Does the baby resemble anyone in the family?
_____
_____
_____

Any other observations?
_____
_____
_____
_____
_____
_____
_____
_____
_____
_____

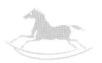

Hospital Records

You are entitled to a copy of the hospital's delivery room notes (doctors' and nurses' comments, anesthetist's records, etc.). Ask your family physician to obtain these for you and insert them here.

_____
_____
_____
_____
_____
_____
_____
_____
_____
_____
_____
_____
_____
_____
_____
_____
_____
_____
_____
_____
_____
_____
_____
_____
_____
_____
_____
_____
_____
_____
_____

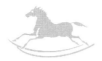

Birth Certificate

Insert one copy here. Keep the other in a safe place.

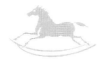

The World on the Day Your Baby was Born

Capture the events and the mood of the country by clipping headlines and short articles from newspapers and magazines. Include politics, entertainment, fashion, sports, lists of best-selling books and records and the horoscope of the day.

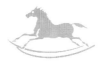

Naming Your Child

Names

_____

These names were chosen because

_____
_____
_____
_____
_____

First portrait of baby

First family picture

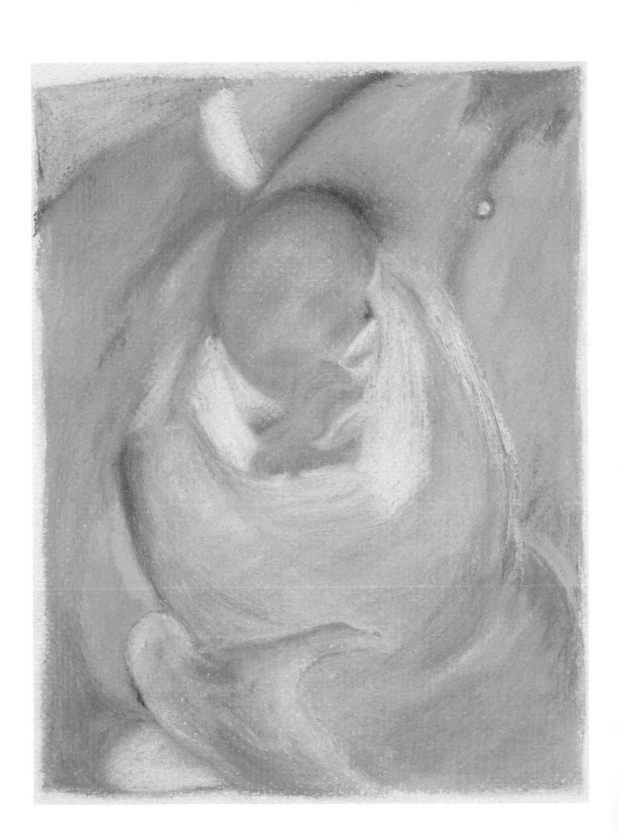

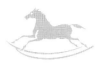

The Newborn

IF THE MOTHER and her baby are fully conscious at birth they will engage in a pattern of behavior which will start with the mother

- smiling at the child
- looking directly into the newborn's face
- holding the child
- embracing the child
- touching her affectionately
- speaking to her affectionately
- offering the breast

The baby in turn will respond by looking, smiling, touching and suckling. Such behavior has been widely accepted as evidence of early post-natal maternal bonding.

Though much work still needs to be done in this area, the basic premise of the bonding theory is simple: the more contact there is immediately after birth between the baby and her parents, the better the outlook for their future relationship.

Bonding is not an absolute and lots of babies born by caesarean section, for example, will grow up just fine even though their mothers were anesthetized when they were born. But in terms of the ideal experience, being close to one's mother and father after birth seems to be a significant positive factor in the development of a loving relationship between the baby and his parents. Therefore, if circumstances permit it, I suggest you breastfeed your baby, have him stay in your room in the hospital and for a few weeks at home. Hug the baby as often as possible and carry him on your body a lot. If you do not breastfeed your baby, hold the bottle while cuddling him in your arms. Never just prop up a bottle and leave him to fend for himself.

Coming Home

Mother and baby came home on

_____

Home was at

_____
_____
_____

How did you travel? Who was with you?

_____
_____
_____

Did either mother or baby have to stay in the hospital? Why?

_____
_____
_____
_____
_____
_____

Are you getting any help with the baby from grandparents, relatives, friends, public health nurses, babysitters?

_____
_____
_____
_____
_____

Describe the first few days at home with your baby.

_____
_____
_____
_____
_____
_____
_____
_____

Does your child have any feeding or sleeping problems?

_____
_____
_____

Do you breastfeed or bottle feed?

_____

How would you describe your baby's personality in the first three months?
What characteristics are strongest?

_____
_____
_____
_____
_____
_____
_____
_____
_____

How would you describe your child's personality at six months of age?

_____
_____
_____
_____
_____
_____
_____
_____
_____
_____

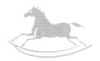

Spiritual or
Religious Ceremonies

Date and type of religious ceremony: circumcision, christening, other

_____
_____
_____
_____
_____

Where was it performed and who was present?

_____
_____
_____
_____
_____
_____
_____
_____
_____
_____
_____
_____
_____
_____
_____

Baby's godfather(s)

_____
_____

Baby's godmother(s)

_____
_____

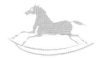

Baby's Room

Describe your baby's nursery in detail and insert a photo of it here.

_____
_____
_____
_____
_____
_____
_____
_____
_____
_____
_____

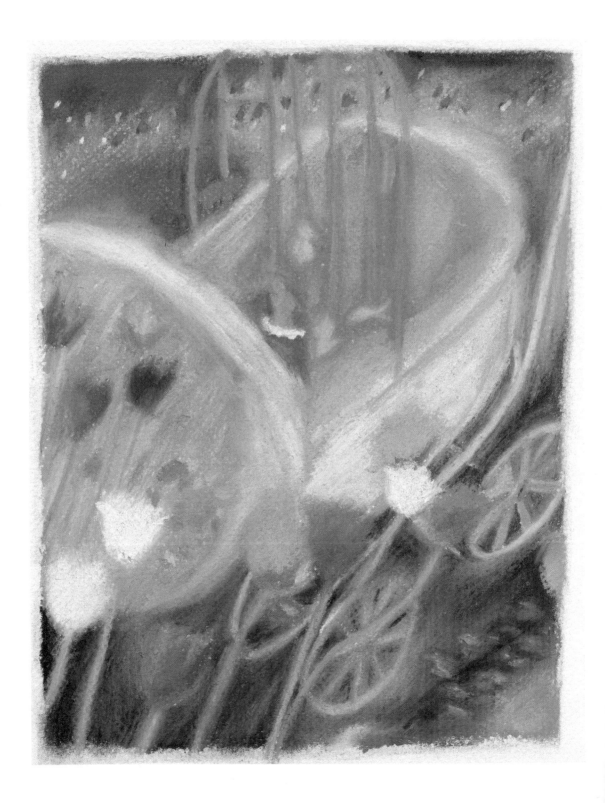

The Incredible Brain
Power of Infants

THE NEWBORN CHILD'S sensory systems are operational from birth on, enabling him to know exactly what is going on around him. Because his expressive faculties, that is, his voice, the movements of his facial muscles, head, arms, hands, etc. are also well under his control, a baby, even during the first days of his life, is a far more discriminating and communicating individual than the thrashing automaton he was depicted to be just a few decades ago.

Professor J.E. Steiner of the Hebrew University in Jerusalem has studied extensively the reaction of infants to taste and smell.[16] In a series of tests he applied sweet, sour and bitter substances to term-born normal infants in the very first hours of life prior to any type of feeding. In every instance sweet stimulation induced facial relaxation and an expression of enjoyment resembling a smile. Sour stimulation led to a typical lip pursing, bitter stimulation to an archlike mouth opening or depressed mouth angles expressive of disgust; and water produced a swallow without facial expression.

When it comes to differentiating smells, babies are probably more competent than adults. This was demonstrated several years ago by Dr. Aidan Macfarlane.[17] He asked nursing mothers to wear gauze pads inside their bras between their feedings. Then he placed its own mother's pad on one side of each infant's head and another mother's pad on the other side. Almost all the infants recognized their mother's pads by turning towards them.

By the age of one week a baby can pick out her mother's voice from a group of other women's voices and at two weeks can recognize that her mother's voice and face belong together. This was demonstrated very elegantly by English researcher Genevieve Carpenter who subjected two-week-old babies to the following situations:

a) mother speaking naturally to her infant
b) another woman speaking naturally to same infant
c) mother imitating the strange woman's voice
d) the stranger trying to speak like baby's mother

The babies paid most attention to their own mother's voice while becoming very upset by the latter two situations—a frightening combination of the familiar and the unfamiliar.[18]

A study conducted to investigate the difference between infants responding to their mothers on closed circuit television as opposed to a videotape recording of their mothers found that the children quickly lost interest in the videotape but kept communicating on closed circuit.

Other experiments have shown that if you place a baby within hearing distance but out of the line of vision of a man and a woman and ask them to speak simultaneously, the newborn will invariably turn toward the woman. According to T. Berry Brazelton of the Children's Hospital Medical Center in Boston, babies pay special attention to their fathers as well.[19] "Amazingly enough," says Brazelton, "when several weeks old, an infant displays an entirely different attitude—more wide-eyed, playful and bright-faced—toward its father than its mother." Brazelton thinks babies perceive their fathers' higher expectations as compared to their mothers' and therefore, respond in more extreme ways.

Children are born with a truly astonishing competence to communicate their needs non-verbally and to tune in to their environments. As two University of Western Ontario psychologists, David Pederson and Greg Moran, have shown, newborns are capable of making all twenty-four separate facial expressions an adult can make. A few weeks after birth they can even learn to control their facial muscles sufficiently to begin to imitate adults.

Mimicry requires the mastery of many sophisticated intellectual skills. Since Jean Piaget, the pioneering child psychologist, other child psychologists have believed that children younger than nine months were incapable of such imitation. But two American psychologists have recently shown that some babies as young as one hour old were able to mimic an experimenter who stuck out his tongue at them, opened his mouth wide or shook his head from side to side. Most babies learn to copy facial expressions at twelve to twenty-two days of age.

This research by Andrew Meltzoff and Keith Moore proves quite convincingly that the infant can respond not only to his bodily needs, but also to emotional messages.[20] In order for the mimicry to take place, the baby has to understand that adults making funny faces will be pleased if the baby imitates them. The baby's only reward for responding in the expected way is a smile and some encouraging words. You could not teach the smartest mouse to run a maze by this approach.

Babies express themselves not only with their facial movements, but also with the rest of their bodies. Two pediatricians, Condon and Sander, filmed adults talking to newborn babies.[21] By slowing down the film they were able to show that the babies' bodies were actually moving to synchronize with the adults' words. Disconnected syllables, random noise or tapping will not elicit this response—only the natural rhythms of speech. Furthermore, children respond the same way whether they are spoken to in English or Chinese. This would strongly suggest that babies, like domestic pets, react to the emotional message—love, caring, indifference, guilt—rather than the meaning of the spoken word.

Babies rarely misinterpret adults' attitudes towards them. The same cannot be said about parents. This subject has now been studied in great depth by various researchers. The best known of these is Daniel Stern at Cornell and author of "The First Relationship: Mother and Infant."[22] His research tool: two videotape cameras running simultaneously. One is trained on the baby's face and the other on the mother's. From watching hours of videotaped infant-mother interactions, one can discern what Stern calls "standard sequences" of behavior.

Some of these are perfectly good and growth-enhancing, others are obviously what one might call "crossed communications." They will leave both participants angry and in the long run, if not corrected, lead to neurotic behavior in the child.

Stern in his book gives many examples of both types of sequences. A positive interaction would consist of mother and infant locking eyes and then moving in synchrony, with the mother speaking to the baby and the baby responding with obvious pleasure until they both calm down, relax and enter a quiet phase.

A negative exchange would be characterized by mother and infant locking eyes as above but then mother shifting all her actions into high gear, making a loud noise, rapidly changing her facial expressions, occasionally shaking the baby, or tossing the baby up in the air until the baby is overwhelmed and finally breaks gaze. The mother fails to interpret this as a signal for her to slow down. Instead, she swings her head around in order to re-establish eye contact with her baby. At this point the infant may start crying or again turn away and mother puts her down wondering what's wrong.

A mother such as the one just described who is having trouble relating to her baby can often be helped in a matter of minutes by watching herself interact with her baby on videotape and having the sequences explained to her.

Today, researchers have discovered an essential element to good baby care: namely, understanding the baby. In Stern's view: "Basic trust that when you're hungry you're going to be fed is clearly important. But I think one of the things that's most basic and important to a baby is being understood. Certainly by the third or fourth month of life, being understood starts to be very important. I can conceive of babies doing reasonably well if feeding is just minimally handled. But they're going to have a lot more trouble if

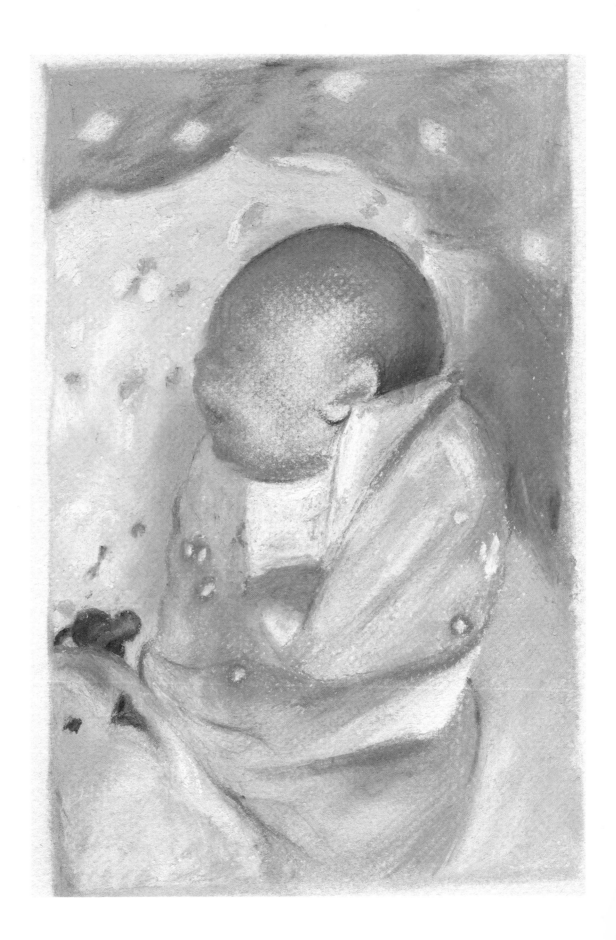

they're not understood."

Parents will enhance their relationships with their babies if they remember that no matter how tiny these children are, they are little people with their own likes and dislikes, personalities and feelings. They are also resilient. There is no need to be overly cautious about what you say or how you behave with them, as long as you remain aware of their essential humanity.

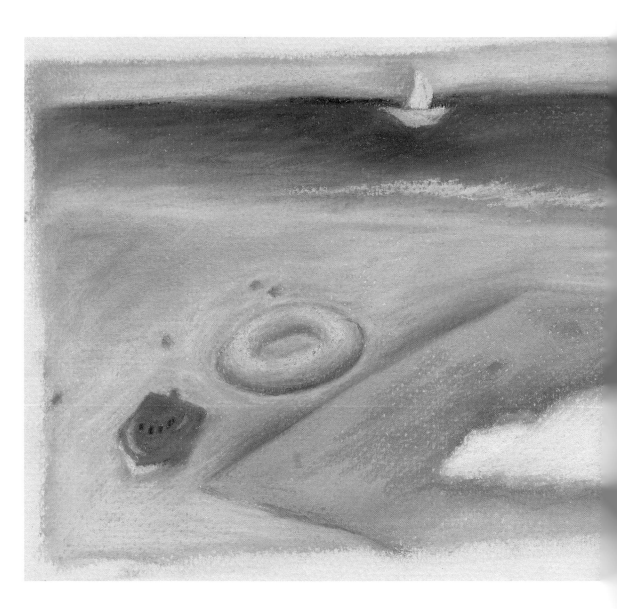

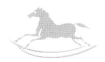

Favorites and Firsts

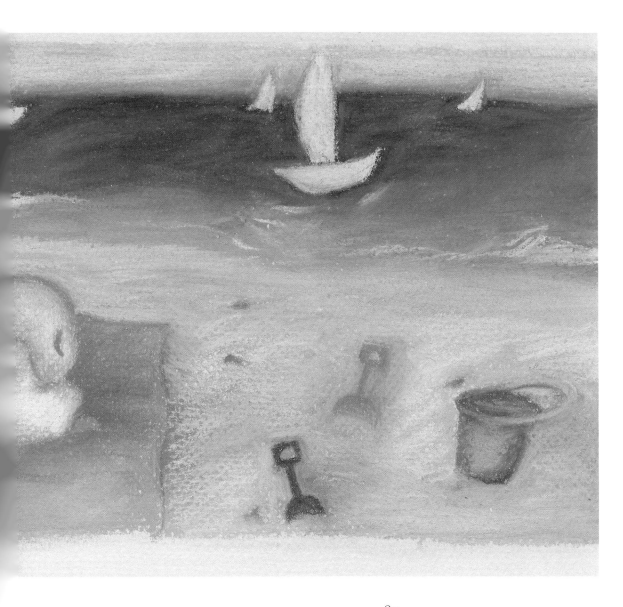

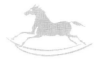

Baby's Favorites

Games

_____
_____
_____
_____

Songs

_____
_____
_____
_____

Exercise

_____
_____
_____
_____

Stories

_____
_____
_____
_____

Toys

_____
_____
_____
_____

Nursery rhymes

_____
_____
_____
_____

Food

_____
_____
_____
_____
_____

Books

_____
_____
_____
_____
_____

Music

_____
_____
_____
_____

Pets

_____
_____
_____
_____

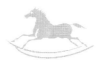

Baby's Memorable "Firsts"

First smile

_____

_____

_____

_____

_____

_____

Rolls over

_____

_____

_____

_____

_____

_____

Sits up

_____

_____

_____

_____

_____

_____

Crawls

_____

_____

_____

_____

_____

_____

Stands up

_____
_____
_____
_____

First visit to doctor

_____
_____
_____
_____

First accident

_____
_____
_____
_____
_____

First illness

_____
_____
_____
_____
_____

First tooth

_____
_____
_____

First friend

_____
_____
_____
_____

First holiday

_____
_____
_____
_____

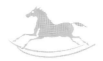

Baby's Weight and Height

	Weight	Height
1st week		
2nd week		
3rd week		
4th week		
2 months		
3 months		
4 months		
6 months		
1 year		

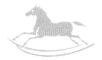

References

1. Rugh, Roberts and Landrum B. Shettles. *From Conception to Birth*. Harper & Row, New York, 1971, p. 61.

2. Wedenberg, E. and B. Johanssen. "When the Fetus Isn't Listening," *Medical World News*. April 10, 1970, pp. 28-29.

3. Liley, Albert W. "The Foetus as a Personality," *Australian and New Zealand Journal of Psychiatry*. 1972, vol. 6(2), pp. 99-105.

4. Walker, D. et al. "The Acoustic Component of the Fetal Environment," *Journal of Reproduction and Fertility*. Jan. 24, 1971, pp. 125-126.

   Grimwade, J.C. et al. "Response of the Human Fetus to Sensory Stimulation," *Australian and New Zealand Journal of Obstetrics and Gynecology*. Nov. 10, 1970, pp. 222-224.

5. Clements, Michele. "Observations on Certain Aspects of Neonatal Behavior in Response to Auditory Stimuli," paper delivered at 5th International Congress of Psychosomatic Obstetrics and Gynecology, Rome, 1977.

6. For a detailed discussion of this subject see *The Secret Life of the Unborn Child* by Thomas R. Verny with John Kelly, Doubleday, Toronto and New York, 1981.

7. DeCasper, Anthony J., and William P. Fifer. "Of Human Bonding: Newborns Prefer Their Mothers' Voices," *Science*. June 6, 1980, vol. 208, pp. 1174-76.

8. Kolata, Gina. "Studying Learning in the Womb," *Science*. July 20, 1984, vol. 225, pp. 302-303.

9. "Human Fetuses Perceive Maternal Speech," *Behavior Today Newsletter*. Feb. 4, 1985, vol. 16(5), pp. 1-7.

10. Ludington-Hoe, Susan, with Susan K. Golant. *How to Have a Smarter Baby*. Rawson Associates, New York, 1985.

11. Armitage, S.E., B.A. Baldwin and M.A. Vince. "The Fetal Sound Environment of Sheep," *Science*. 1980, vol. 208(6), pp. 1171-1174.

12. Bench, R.J., J.H. Anderson and M. Hoare. "Measurement System for Fetal Audiometry," *Journal of the Acoustical Society of America*. 1970, vol. 47, pp. 1602-1606.

13. Bernard, J. and L.W. Sontag. "Fetal Reactivity to Tonal Stimulation: A Preliminary Report," *Journal of Genetic Psychology*. 1947, vol. 70, pp. 205-210.

    Bernholz, J.C. and B.R. Benacerraf. "The Development of Human Fetal Hearing," *Science*. 1983, vol. 222(4), pp. 516-518.

14. Shetler, Donald J. "Prenatal Music Experiences," *Music Education Journal*. March 1985, vol. 71(7), pp. 26-27.

15. Winget, Carolyn, and Frederick Kapp, "The Relationship of the Manifest Content of Dreams to Duration of Labor in Premiparae," *Psychosomatic Medicine*. July-Aug. 1972, pp. 313-319.

16. Steiner, J.E. "Facial Expressions of the Neonate Infant Indicating the Hedonics of Food Related Chemical Stimuli," in Weiffenbach, J.M. (ed.), *Taste and Development: The Genesis of Sweet Preference*. U.S. Government Printing Office, Washington, D.C., 1977.

17. Macfarlane, Aidan. "Olfaction in the Development of Social Preferences in the Human Neonate," *Parent-Infant Interaction*. Paper delivered at CIBA Symposium #33, Associated Scientific Publishers, Inc., New York, 1975.

18. Restak, Richard M. "Newborn Knowledge," *Science*. June 1982, pp. 23-28.

19. Ibid.

20. Meltzoff, Andrew N. and M. Keith Moore. *The Origins of Imitation In Infancy: Paradigm, Phenomena, and Theories*. Ablex Publishing Corporation, Norwood, N.J., 1983.

21. Condon, S.W. and L.W. Sander. "Neonate Movement is Synchronized with Adult Speech: Interaction Participation and Language Acquisition," *Science*. 1974, pp. 99-101.

22. Stern, Daniel. "A Micro-Analysis of Mother-Infant Interaction," *Journal of American Academy of Child Psychiatry*. 1971, vol. 10(3).

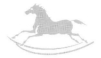

Baby Chart

How to tell what your baby is doing physically and mentally from conception to birth.

Month	Week	Day	Size and Weight	Embryological Changes	Functional Development
1	1	2	Microscopic	4-8 cells.	9 days—HCG—human chorionic gonado-tropin is produced. Pregnancy test based on this.
		3		16-32 cells, raspberry shaped ball—morula.	
		5		A hollow sphere—blastocyst, consists of about 150 cells.	
	2	7	1/100 in., 1/3 mm	Implantation occurs 7-9 days after conception. 1/3 to 1/2 of all fertilized ova die during the first month.	
		12		Embryo has embedded itself into lining of uterus, placenta begins to form, yolk sac appears.	
	3	18		Anchoring villi develop, the nervous system begins to develop.	
		20	1/16 in., 1.8 mm	The foundation for the child's brain, spinal cord and peripheral nervous system and rudiments of the eyes are formed; first blood vessels appear, heart delineated.	
	4	28	1/4 in., 7 mm = the diameter of a standard lead pencil	Building blocks for 40 pairs of muscles develop, 33 pairs of vertebrae appear, blood vessels proliferate, heart begins to beat, body now consists of a head, a trunk, a tail and tiny arm buds, the mouth first opens, placenta fully functional.	Mouth opens on the 28th day for the first time; slow, generalized movements of head, trunk and extremities evoked by stimuli to the skin.
2	5	35	1/3 in., 10 mm 1/1000 oz., 2.8 mg	The three primary parts of the brain are present, as are all cranial nerves and spinal nerves, eyes, ears and nose have started to form, eye pigment present, outer ear with auditory canal develops, arm buds and leg buds prominent, heart cavity develops chambers, the digestive tract, spleen and pancreas are formed, umbilical cord fully established.	
	6	42	1/2 in., 13 mm	Eyes become pigmented, tip of nose, rudiments of fingers and toes appear, the thalamus (major relay center of the brain), the hypothalamus and cerebellum are formed, certain reflex pathways are established, septation of heart complete, muscles are lengthening, cartilage and bones develop, testes and ovaries appear. After 6 weeks called a fetus.	The earliest reflexes begin; sucking and grasping; heart is incomplete but pumping blood. ECG's similar to those of adult; fetus responds to touch with large generalized movements; strong and brisk spontaneous fetal movements appear.
	7		4/5 in., 2 cm	Face rounds out and begins to look human, a distinct neck connects the head with the body. The semi-circular canals of the ear, the palate of the mouth and heart valves form, the nerve cells of the retina, corpus striatum and thalamus develop, cortical synapses appear.	Responds to tactile stimulation.

Month	Week	Size and Weight	Embryological Changes	Functional Development	Psychological Development
	8	1-1/4 in., 3 cm 1/30 oz., 1 g Diameter of a 50-cent piece, lighter than a Valium tablet	The eyes have moved to the front, taste buds in the mouth begin to form, the head comprises about half the fetus; stomach big, arms and legs small, subcortical synapses appear.	Light stroking of upper lip or wings of the nose will cause bending of the neck and trunk away from the source of stimulation; moves head, arms, trunk easily. EEG tracings show brain activity similar to that of adults.	
	9	1-1/2 in., 3.7 cm 1/7 oz., 4 g	Teeth are beginning to develop, as do fingernails, toenails and hair follicles; the skin becomes thicker; the skeleton and all the muscles are rapidly growing; nerves supplying the eyes, the nose, the tongue and the vestibular system for balance are all in place; males form a penis, females a uterus and vagina.	When the eyelids or the palms of the hands are touched they both react by closing; the fetus does not jerk its entire body back as it did earlier; responds to changes in position of its mother.	
3	10	2-1/8 in., 5.3 cm 1/4 oz., 7 g	The palate closes, muscles of the digestive tract functional, gall bladder secretes bile, lungs complete, external genitalia well defined, the brain organized along adult lines.	If the forehead is touched, the fetus will turn its head away.	
	12	3 in., 7.5 cm 1/2 oz., 14 g The weight of an ordinary letter.	Taste buds morphologically mature, olfactory nerve (smell) fully developed, lungs begin to expand and contract regularly, thumb can be opposed to the forefinger, all of its major systems are formed and the baby is virtually a functioning organism.	Can kick, turn its feet, curl its toes, frown, purse its lips, swallow some amniotic fluid. If its lips are stroked, the fetus will respond by sucking.	Unborn children of the same age begin to show individual variations particularly evident in facial expressions.
4	16	6 in., 15 cm 4 oz., 112 g	Period of maximum growth. Fetal heart fully developed; pulse rate is about 120-160 beats a minute; eyes become sensitive to light; surface of the brain forms many convolutions. Spinal nerves and roots acquire myelin. Fetal skeleton detectable on X-ray.	Baby will react to a bitter substance (iodine) in the amniotic fluid by ceasing to drink it and by frowning; to a sweet substance (saccharine) by doubling its normal rate of ingestion. It will react to cold fluids and to tickling. Shine a light on mother's abdomen and baby will shield its eyes; make a loud noise and it will cover its ears.	Begins to suck thumb (for comfort?). Grasps umbilical cord; likelihood of capability for conditioned learning and therefore rudimentary memory, intentional behavior.
	18		Youngest known child that has survived premature birth, Marcus Richardson of Cincinnati was born in 1971, 18 weeks after conception.	Fetal hiccup audible and visible through the abdominal wall.	Brain life manifest.
5	20	8 in., 20 cm	Hearing apparatus complete; hands develop a strong grip; crying patterns of prematurely born babies identifiable as related to their mothers' voice prints. Myelination in neck region of spinal cord.	Baby kicks and turns; occasionally may hiccup or cry audibly; sensitive as any one-year-old to touch; will react to music or loud noise.	Periods of drowsiness and sleep alternate with periods of activity. Discriminates differences in sound.
	24	10-12 in., 25-30 cm	Now a miniature human being, more than doubles its weight. Eyelids open, feeble respiratory movements begin.	Pupilary response.	Begins to dream, listens attentively; keyed to mother's heartbeat; adults recall memories from 6 months on, though hard to pinpoint. Violent shifts of body or kicking / Variations in heartbeat / Unusual loss or gain of weight / Too much thumb sucking } Indicative of unborn's discomfort or experience of stress.

Month	Week	Size and Weight	Embryological Changes	Functional Development	Psychological Development
6	28	12 in., 30 cm 2-3 lb., 1-1 1/2 kg	Cerebral hemispheres expand enormously and large convolutions develop, six cortical layers formed. All reflexes evident at birth already present; i.e., sucking, rooting, moro, grasp and step reflexes.	Will respond to sweet, sour or acrid substances placed on its tongue by changing facial expression. Preemie will respond differentially to smells.	Moves in rhythm to music, shows preferences in music; twins may react differently to the same piece of music; conditioned learning demonstrable; able to discriminate substances by taste and smell; will signal displeasure by vigorous kicking; "plays" with parents through abdominal wall.
7	32	13 in., 32.5 cm Sitting position. 4-5 lb. 2-2 1/2 kg	Most of its weight gain consists of fat deposited under the skin; eyelids no longer fused; eyebrows and hair on head appear. Synergy established between right and left cerebral hemispheres, myelinization of brain begins.	Skin is functioning efficiently to protect baby against heat loss. Could survive now with relative ease outside of the womb.	Reacts differently to voices of mother, father and unknown people.
8	36	14-15 in., 35-37.5 cm in sitting position. 19-20 in., 47.5-50 cm in overall length. 6-8 lb. 3-3 1/2 kg	Assumes an upside-down position. Skin is pink. Fingernails and toenails formed.	Less active than previously because of cramped quarters.	Mentally ready to engage the world

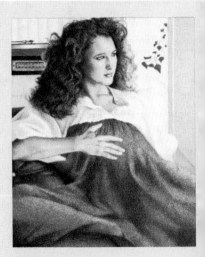